Benzodiazepine and Seroquel Hell: A Guide to
Getting Off of These Poisons

By Young Kim

Dedicated to A.R. and my family, whose love, inspiration, and support allowed me to write.

Printed in the United States of America

First Printing, 2016

ISBN

Young Kim

7817 N. Oconto Ave

Niles, IL 60714

youngkim3000@yahoo.com

Table of Contents

Introduction

Introduction

A long time ago, back in 2001, I entered graduate school at the University of Illinois for a degree in medicine. The tests and workload were beyond anything that I had imagined. I couldn't imagine how stressful it was! I was not prepared for it. I had always been so studious and did extremely well in school. I had attended the University of Chicago and graduated with high honors. As such, I felt I was unstoppable. Unfortunately, as I read over all the credentials of my classmates, I discovered that all of them were just as smart as I was.

After being so utterly anxious for the first few months, I went to see my family doctor and explained my feelings. I suppose with sincere intentions, he tried to help me. He prescribed for me something called Klonopin which is part of the benzodiazepine family of medicines. They are called anxiolytics and are supposed to help with nervousness and sleep problems (both of which I had experienced). I felt I needed help in both areas, so my family doctor who was double boarded in Psychiatry prescribed them to me. Little would I know that it would be the end of my life as I knew it. I will forever remember the day as the critical juncture of my life which turned my life upside down.

When I went home that day, I took one of the tablets which was blue, and put it under my tongue. Immediately, I felt a dizziness come over me. After about two minutes, I felt so tired and lethargic. I was stumbling and losing my balance. Within five minutes, I collapsed asleep, and fell into one of the deepest sleep episodes of my entire life. As I was very young and sort of ignorant, I thought the medicine was working so great. All my anxiety disappeared! Also, I felt like I found some kind of magic sleeping potion which would allow me to take naps instantly after a long night of studying and before I went to bed. I felt that it would be more "efficient" and this medicine would give me more control over my time to manage in medical school (because I could fall asleep instantly), which I was always in short supply of. In addition, I thought I could take a pill before exams which would lessen my anxiety.

Little did I know (hindsight is always 20/20) that I would be sealing my grave with respect to my studies. My memory faded quickly (something obviously essential in medical school), and I also quickly built up a tolerance that made me have to consume more and more pills as the weeks passed. I also started to have other terrible side effects, like "benzo rage" and driving problems (I got into a few car accidents during this time). Soon, I was taking the pills every day in larger numbers. After a year and a half, I had to change doctors and temporarily ran out of pills for a period of a week. Then, the ultimate nightmare started...

I remember the night it happened. I was without the pills for about 3 days, and I strangely found that I could not fall asleep for the life of me! I tossed and turned and stayed up the entire night. As the next day wore on, my anxiety grew and grew until I felt I was going to have a nervous breakdown. The following night, I tried to drink a glass of wine to relax, but it was of no use. And I was so wide awake! Even though I had a hard day at the hospital, I could not sleep a wink! It was intractable insomnia. I quickly did some Internet searches, and I stumbled upon what I was facing. I learned quickly that I had done some serious near permanent damage to my brain. I was to face "Benzodiazepine Withdrawal Syndrome".

I suffering several more nights of no sleep, and I started to panic. After finding another doctor, I went back on the benzodiazepines, and slowly got back to the doses I was on before. However, shortly afterward, I decided to get off of the medicines. It was just too intolerable to go through medical school and face the side effects which made studying so difficult.

But those horrible benzodiazepines would not let me off so easily. I tried to taper off, and my brain and body got worse and worse. I had to ask for a leave of absence from medical school due to the suffering I was enduring. The next year was spent in the worst suffering I had ever imagined. When I complained about this, my new doctor prescribed to me Seroquel to use to taper off the Klonopin. That was just substituting one problem for another. With Seroquel, I also had the difficult issue of weight gain.

I made a conscious decision that no matter what, I would get off of these drugs from Hell. During this torture-fest, I read about how many people felt getting off of either Benzodiazepines and/or Seroquel was harder than any other addiction or experience they encountered. Many argued that it was more painful than the greatest torture, more addictive than heroin or crack cocaine...

The withdrawal from both of those medications were beyond a hellish realm that I couldn't have even imagined up, even in my wildest dreams. The pain that I endured was so great that I contemplated suicide so many times. But there is a happy ending. After many trials, I finally freed myself from this hell realm.

I am writing this book to share my story of suffering, and to report that as of today, I have been free of benzodiazepines for many years. I want to share a story of hope that one can be free of these awful medications, but it will take some great patience, courage, determination, willpower, knowledge, and prayer. It will also take a drastic change in how to live your life so that you will not need those medications to alleviate your psychological suffering.

I hope that anyone reading this book would be free someday of these dangerous and terrible drugs, and understand how disgusting they are. The drugs are not natural, and usually only serve to make your problems even worse. For a select minority, such medications may be necessary, but in my opinion there are far better methods to tackle the problems in your life than to ingest such poisons into your system. Once they are in your system, they will slowly change your physical brain chemistry to completely depend on them, and when you find yourself without them, your mind and body will go into a desperate panic and this will in turn make your life into a living hell. I will chronicle what I believe is the road back to finding your own inner strength and freedom from these toxic drugs.

Chapter 1: This is How You Got Hooked

If you are reading this, then you are probably sick and tired of being addicted to benzodiazepines and Seroquel. You were probably given a diagnosis of anxiety, bipolar disorder, or insomnia. There are other uses like for muscle relaxation, pre-surgery, or seizures, or alcohol withdrawal. But most likely you were going through a rough period and wanted something to calm or chill you out. So you went to your doctor and asked for help. He gave you benzodiazepines or Seroquel.

Benzodiazepines, in the name of Xanax, Valium, Klonopin, or Ativan (among others), work by changing the effect of a neurotransmitter called gamma aminobutyric acid or GABA. Seroquel works on the dopamine and serotonin (5HT) receptors and is classified as an antipsychotic. There can be many uses for both in the psychiatric world, which I believe grossly overmedicates people. Personally, I think people need to use every other possible way to either recover from their anxiety or insomnia (or any other crazy notions) before they turn to these odious poisons, which is basically a one-way street to Hell.

I think one of the major problems with mental health and the health care system in general is that everyone is looking for a quick and easy fix. Instead of trying to either meditate, or exercise, or pray, or just learn to cope, or find a way to remove yourself from the stressor, most people (with their doctors in support) choose to take a pill to solve their problems. This is a giant mistake.

The problem is that once you start messing with the body and the brain, you are wreaking havoc to what nature has been building for billions of years. If you are under stress, mentally or physically, that is the body's innate wisdom telling you to STOP THAT BEHAVIOR that is messing up your life! If you are living with a crazy boyfriend/girlfriend, and you are stressed, you need to work on that or leave. If you are in graduate school like I was and stressed out beyond belief, then you need to either just cope or withdraw from school. What you don't do is attempt to fix everything magically with a pill. It never works. In my case, it destroyed my mind, my sleep patterns, my memory, my physical reaction times (I got into car accidents), and so many relationships.

Doctors don't mind prescribing these highly addictive drugs because it is a quick fix for them too. They don't have to sit down and listen for so long about your personal problems. They also get to write a new prescription a month and see you at their office monthly upon which they will bill you a nice day's wage of yours for the cost of the refill appointment. Ten minutes of their time (asking if you are doing ok on the meds), in exchange for a day or two of your labor.

The Big Pharma companies love them too because they are so highly addictive. Once someone gets hooked on them, they are usually a customer for life. So you will see ads for these toxic poisons on your television, in your magazines, and on your computer screen. The side effects are often intolerable, and if you try to come off of them you will be faced with the worst withdrawal symptoms imaginable.

Chapter 2: Listen to These Withdrawal Stories of Hell

First of all, I want to emphasize that you are going to be completely unaware of just how harmful these poisonous "medicines" (which are just another set of addictive drugs) are until it is too late. They will seem to work as intended—at first. Your anxiety will lessen, or you will be able to sleep better.   Then slowly, insidiously, they will start to show its terrible side effects.   There are so many (excessive grogginess in the morning, dizziness, weight gain, memory loss, etc.) that will become very bothersome and then simply intolerable.

After you have built up a tolerance and are taking more and more of the pills months later, you will realize that you are completely hooked and addicted. You will panic when you are running low in your medicine bottle. You will feel desperate when you forgot your medicines at home and you find yourself away at a friend's house.

With your newfound assessment that these medicines are just dangerous drugs, you may change your mind and want off of them. You think you can just quit and stop taking them. You think it will be easy. But you are wrong. Like a cancer, they have spread their evil through your body. Recovery will be long and painful.   The withdrawal period will now begin. If you were lucky and decided to quit early, then the suffering of withdrawal will be short. But for many who did not catch on early (myself included), recovery will be long and protracted.

Withdrawal from Benzodiazepines (and I am including Seroquel too since it is often prescribed in a similar fashion with similar side effects), will be Hell. Pure Hell... Just face it now. I am not being pessimistic. I am just being realistic. This type of thinking will actually make it paradoxically easier because you will have to brace yourself and find the strength to overcome.

As you find yourself in Hell, it will help IMMENSELY (as it did for me), read and read and read some more about others who are suffering just like you. Knowing you are not alone makes your suffering much more tolerable. Now, I just wanted to insert a few withdrawal stories here that would indicate that you are not alone. There are millions of people addicted to any one of the benzodiazepines and Seroquel (and other similar drugs). Just to represent them in their own words, I did not correct for grammar and spelling. Once again, these are not side effects per se, but we are talking about the withdrawal symptoms once you either stop cold turkey or start reducing your dosage. From the website blog:

http://www.crazyboards.org/forums/index.php?/topic/62359-coming-off-seroquel-hell/

lauraishere

- Member
-

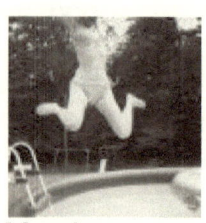

-
- Member
-

- 92 posts

Posted 6 Feb 2013 (edited)

This is terrible! Just need a place to complain. I haven't been to sleep and it's 7:30 here, in part due to the nasuea and in part, probably, due to the lack of drug. I did everything responsibly and slowly with the psychiatrist, tapered ever so slowly over a matter of 3 or so months from 100 to 50 to 25, and then even tried to break that 25 in half...but still, I am getting this terrible "withdrawl." I just need to wait it out so the drug can finally get out of my system, because everytime I try I cave to the nasuea and take more. I'm even trying to get someone to cover my shift bc i feel so sick...ugh, what a stupid reason to miss work.

Did/is anyone else having as terrible a time coming off of this drug as me?

saoirse

- "seer-sha"
-

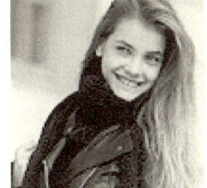

-
- Member
-
- 485 posts
- Gender:Woman

Posted 6 Feb 2013

15

Coming off of Seroquel was hell, at least until the hypomania set in. Then I was briefly euphoric. But yeah, it's one of the rougher drugs I've come off of, especially given that my old pdoc was a moron and had me stop it cold turkey.

lauraishere

enlightened_plutonium, you seem like me... going for my second night fully w/o it on 0 hours of sleep. naseau still present. i am DETERMINED to get off this stuff. seems like heroin withdrawl would be easier lol

MiaB

- another crazy cat person
-

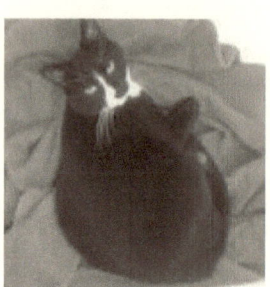

-
- Inmate
- ★★   Staff
-
-
- 5661 posts
- Gender:female

Posted 7 Feb 2013

Totally understand - I wound up in the ER on a drip and heavy duty anti nausea meds when coming off

16

seroquel suddenly. The withdrawal is a complete bitch. You need to watch out for dehydration, and if you haven't already, I strongly advise you to ask your pdoc for a prescription strength antiemetic to control the nausea.

Seroquel is actually a part of my current med cocktail, and while I believe it's the most helpful drug I'm on, I feel that after my discontinuation experiences, I'm pretty much trapped now and will be on it for life.

Kid Amine 26-11-2012, 03:12

I'm here again, this time to warn about Seroquel (Quietiapine). This last week has been pure hell, like a Twilight Zone episode. To wit: Last Saturday, I visited a friend. Told her of me and my fiances' sleep problems. She gave me a load of 300mg seroquels, probably a dozen or so. I was most grateful, even tho I hate this shit, its better than chronic insomnia. That is, until Sunday morning. I was fine, aside from the HORRID drymouth and munchies. My fiance, however, was NOT fine. She was.... how can I put it... had a full reality break with paranoid delusions. Talking all kinds of crazy shit for FOUR DAYS. She talked like her dead grandma. She thought she was in the show "Mad Men", working as an advertising consultant. She accused me of spending all her money, she flushed her meds down the drain thinking they were implants out to get her, she tried to smoke a pen thinking it was a cigarette, tried to operate the Wii with a notepad, the list goes on, Finally, on Thursday, she was mostly quiet, and talked none of the nonsense of the past few days. She seems okay now. I ruled out seizure, stroke, aneurism, or me being the one who was psychotic. I dont know if anyone has seen anything like this before. She has taken Seroquel before, hell, she was on 600mg/day for a year before she got off of it (due to massive weight gain). This is the first time with ANY drug that I would physically restrain someone (her) from taking again if it came to that. My question is this: does anyone know wtf happened? I was thinking serotonin syndrome, but even that doesnt explain this. I swear another few days of that and I would have had to commit her. Far scarier than an OD.

This is a story of Benzodiazepine Withdrawal from the website

http://www.benzo.org.uk/barry.htm

BARRY HASLAM'S STORY

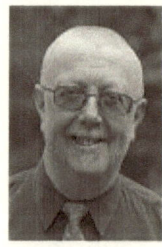

Oldham Tranx · APPGITA Main Page

"A full public inquiry is urgently called for, so those guilty for 40 years of cover up, deaths and misery, can be brought to justice"

In 1976, Barry had a complete mental breakdown after 3 years of intensive studying for his accountancy exams (which he passed with flying colours).

Prior to this, Barry was a loving husband and father to his wife, Sue and daughter, Susan and Katherine (then aged 7 and 6 years).

He was a very fit young man who played competitive football twice a week for many years and had trained/played with professional footballers. He went fishing, for personal tranquillity. These activities stopped for ever after being prescribed benzodiazepines drugs from 1976 to 1986. He was legally prescribed a cocktail of antidepressants and benzodiazepines drugs. In 1981, he was given 10mg. of Ativan daily, then 20mg, and by January 1985, he was on 30mg daily plus 12 tablets daily of strong painkillers for headaches.

By this time, Barry had become violent and very aggressive. His weight had ballooned by 5 stones, and he had become, what he describes as a "sick and evil" person – a Jeckyl and Hyde.

He then experienced a "window of lucidity" when he was able to see himself and what his addiction was doing to his family. He weaned himself of the drugs at home, over a 14 month period and finally on 19 March 1986, he finally became drug free.

Barry says he would not like any other human being to experience the horrors and nightmares of his withdrawal, and his 10 years of complete memory loss due to benzodiazepine neuro-poisoning drugs.

(The facts quoted from 1976 - 1986, have been taken from his wife, Sue and later from his medical records.)

In 1987, he "set off on a trek" to help others, seek the truth on benzodiazepine drugs, and uncover the wall of silence which the medical profession, drug companies and successive Governments have helped to create.

During this time, he found God (or he says God found him) and His love and support. His wife, Sue and now grown up daughters and grandchildren have sustained and nourished his aim for the truth to be known world wide, of the horrors of these drugs.

Fourteen years off the drugs, Barry still suffers from the after effects of the drugs including the following: brain damage, cognitive defects, headaches, partial deafness in both ears, intense pain in right leg (knee to toe), mood swings, circulation problems, hypothyroidism and breathing problems.

In 1996, Barry was the first person in the United Kingdom to receive Disability Living Allowance (DLA) awarded to him by the Department of Social Security's Tribunal Board because of the brain damage caused by benzodiazepines prescribed in large quantities.

It is largely through Barry's persistence and the support and backing of his local Member of Parliament, Phil Woolas, that the "Beat the Benzos" campaign was launched.

Barry says, "a full public inquiry is urgently called for, so those guilty for 40 years of cover up, deaths and misery, can be brought to justice."

On February 24, 1994 David Blunkett MP (then Shadow Secretary of State for Health) in a letter to Barry Haslam about benzodiazepine tranquillisers wrote:

"I am passing your letter to Paul Boateng who, as legal affairs spokesman, has specific responsibility for the litigation side of what is a national scandal."

On February 25, 1994 Paul Boeteng MP also wrote to Barry Haslam and said:

"Clearly, the aim of all involved in this sorry affair is the provision of justice for the victims of these drugs."

Here is another story about someone named Rose, from the website:

http://psychrights.org/Stories/TRAP.htm

on a website for T.R.A.P. (The tranquilizer and Recovery Place). This a good website for recovery support from benzodiazepines and the z drugs.

Benzos and SSRIs: Partners in crime – Rose's story

Here my story. I hope someday I will be able to finish my story with the magic "happily ever after". It doesn't have this ending yet, but I am through the worst and recovering.

I am the mother of three school age kids. I am a doctor and before my encounter with prescription drugs I had a great but sometimes stressful job in Public Health.

My troubles started when I injured my back. I was in constant pain and my doctor prescribed Codeine and NSAIDS. I never really liked drugs so after a while I started taking the Codeine only in the mornings and relying on heat packs in the evenings at home. I lost my appetite, felt nauseated a lot of the time and started losing weight. My sleep became difficult (at least I thought it was difficult but compared to what happened later it was not a big problem!)

I thought I had depression: I have a family history of depression and so I was programmed to think I could suffer it too. Now, I can see that my symptoms could well have been due to NSAIDS and Codeine dependence with interdose withdrawal. NSAIDS like Voltaren which I was on are well known for causing all kinds of digestive problems. Codeine has a half-life of only 2-3 hours so by bedtime each day I would have been in withdrawal. Trouble sleeping is a Codeine withdrawal symptom.

My back specialist told me to stop Codeine as he was worried how long I'd been taking it. He said it was "mind altering". I was really quite shocked as I thought Codeine was safe. I had never heard that Codeine could be addictive. I stopped it cold turkey. My sleep got worse and I was feeling weird but still I didn't think of Codeine withdrawal as being a possible cause.

One night I couldn't sleep and was stressing over a big presentation I had to do at work in the morning. My husband called a mental health line. He is now very sorry he did this and says he panicked. He didn't know it was a *mental* health line. It was just the number the after hours medical centre gave him for someone to talk to. Anyway I ended up with an appointment to see a psychiatrist who put me on Lexapro, Zopiclone and Clonazepam. The psychiatrist never even asked if I had recently changed my pain meds.

I wasn't very happy to start taking benzos, but the psychiatrist said I would only be on Zopiclone and Clonazepam for a few weeks at most while the SSRI had time to work. He claimed SSRIs are so good it would be like a light going on. He also said that one in three people should be on medication for depression. This seemed a bit extreme but he appeared to be a nice guy and so we trusted him. Unfortunately his predictions about Lexapro were completely wrong.

Instead of feeling better I felt worse, much worse. I got agitated and anxious and couldn't sleep even with the benzos. Anxiety and insomnia are well known side effects of SSRIs. What did the psychiatrist do? You guessed it . . . upped the dose of all three drugs. By now I was in little short of a toxic delirium. My heart

23

beat was irregular, my vision was blurred, I had constant migraine and I was shaking and sweating all over. At times my body seemed frozen and I could not move. I was finding it difficult to speak. I could barely stand and couldn't count to ten. I was incapable of the simplest task.

The psychiatrist's only response was more drugs! He told me that it was far better to over treat than under treat and he would just give me more and more and bigger doses until it worked. I think I had 10 drugs in all, up to 4 at a time over a period of only a few months. Some of the other drugs I was prescribed were Halcion, Temazepam, Imipramine and Quetiapine: all given to help me sleep. I remember one occasion when handing me a script he said, "If someone else saw this script they might think I am trying to kill you." Yes, this is a verbatim quote!

All my complaints about how much worse the drugs had made me were ignored. I was constantly told that my mental health was the problem. Yes, I was worse than before starting treatment, but that was going to happen anyway and the drugs were helping me. I became suicidal as I believed that I was severely mentally ill and felt as if every one would be better off if I was dead. Because of my upbringing my attitude to mental illness was very negative. My husband could not leave me alone for a minute. In fact I was told that questioning if my problems had been made worse by drugs was evidence of "disordered thinking", which is in effect only one step away from "thought disorder" i.e. psychosis. More than once I was threatened with admission against my will and only avoided it by lying and saying I was feeling better.

Eventually one mental health nurse listened and got an opinion from a pharmacologist at the local hospital who said my problems could be pharmacological. He advised that the Lexapro dose should be dropped down to the standard dose. Once I dropped the Lexapro dose I improved a bit, the suicidal urges stopped and my husband could go back to work. However I experienced severe SSRI withdrawal including all over body tingling, hot sweats and derealisation even though I was still on the standard dose. I would not have survived this without the information supplied in Dr Healy's article http://www.benzo.org.uk/healy.htm which by then my husband had found.

The psychiatrist I was seeing denied withdrawal was even possible since I was still taking Lexapro and very soon after that (about a week) said he couldn't look after me any more. I was "atypical" and he had no more ideas. He hoped someone else would be able to help me. At least he did seem genuinely sorry for the state I had been left in. He offered to refer me to another psychiatrist but by now my husband and I had lost all faith in psychiatrists and we said no thanks that we would go back to our family doctor.

I decided to stop all the drugs and with a very rapid taper and on my own over about two weeks I did. I experienced severe withdrawal symptoms including diarrhoea, abdominal pains, hot sweats, hypoglycaemia, panic attacks, muscle jerks and of course terrible insomnia and fatigue. In the first few weeks my total sleep hours in a week were often less than 14. I would go 3 nights without any sleep at all. Twice I collapsed on the side of road when out walking. Even so I felt better in withdrawal than while taking the drugs and had a better level of functioning!

After about 3 months off drugs my family doctor sent me to see another psychiatrist for a one off review as I still experiencing severe insomnia and struggling to get through the days. He (the new psychiatrist) seemed to think all my problems were anxiety. He ignored benzo and SSRI withdrawal as possible causes for my ongoing sleeplessness and poor level of functioning. The one good thing that came out of this appointment it was that he said I did not have depression and let my doctor know this. Also good was that he did not suggest any more drug treatment.

I tried many insomnia cures over the first few months (about 40) all of which were ineffective. I also went to another doctor who does hypnotherapy to try and treat my insomnia but it didn't work and in the end he said I should go back on Zopiclone. My own doctor thought so too as she was adamant I could not be withdrawal after 5 months, and said she would prescribe as many Zopiclone tablets as I wanted. I could just phone for a script and she would let all the nurses know not to question me. My husband travels for work and so in desperation I did try a Zopiclone tablet one night: it just did nothing. I slept less than 2 hours and spent the next day crying.

This was a valuable turning point for me. My tolerance to Zopiclone proved I was still in withdrawal. Tolerance and withdrawal are both reflections of drug caused changes in your brain. I saw that my doctor and the psychiatrist I had recently seen did not know the true length of Zopiclone/Clonazepam withdrawal. I decided to find out for myself and come across Dr Ashton's paper on protracted benzodiazepine withdrawal symptoms, http://www.benzo.org.uk/manual/bzcha03.htm with insomnia listed as up to 12 months. Another addiction expert Dr Seven Melemis http://www.addictionsandrecovery.org/benzodiazepine.htm says 2 years. This gave me hope. I knew that my problems were not the result of mental illness but of drug withdrawal and that I would improve with time. I have come to accept that nothing but time will cure me. Even fear is part of the journey and I have to accept it and survive one night and one day at a time.

Since then I have been in recovery. It is now 3 months since I took any Zopiclone and 10 months out from Lexapro. I still have insomnia with lots of myoclonic jerks, sometimes up to 15 times a night, but I have now started to dream again which I feel is a sign of recovery.

The SSRI has damaged the nerves in my feet which are painful, often swell, sweat and go red. It is a peripheral neuropathy and I don't know if it will get better or not. My hands too are affected but to a lesser degree.

I sometimes blame myself for not knowing better as a health worker, but the truth is I had been fed a constant diet of pro drug propaganda. I was completely unaware of what SSRIs can do.

I have lost my job but I do still have my home and family and my back is ok now too. I am often very very tired but once I am well I would love to travel to see Dr Healy, Dr Ashton, Dr Melemis and Dr Breggin to thank them for saving my life by providing truth about these drugs.

Still not sleeping but glad to be alive,
Rose

UPDATE

It is now 20 months since my rapid withdrawal. Slowly and with many ups and downs I have continued to heal. My insomnia is intermittent rather than constant now and I expect to heal more and more as time goes by. The myoclonic jerks are all but gone. My husband and I have continued to learn about the fraudulent promotion and the toxic nature of most psychiatric drugs and we are active in efforts to publicise the d`1angers. I can be contacted at epirose@gmail.comepirose@gmail.com.

I could fill hundreds and thousands of pages detailing the stories of poor unfortunate souls, but I will include just the above stories so you can get a sample of the kind of misery that exists/has existed due to this dangerous psychoactive medications. Please read them yourself to know about the disease you have now contracted. Awareness and understanding is a key for recovery.

Chapter 3: They Did Not Warn Us About Side Effects

If you are in the midst of a terrible ordeal, take a moment to consider if you were even told of the side effects. Yes, they may have told you briefly, but did they really tell you how terrible and extensive they may really be?

(Source
http://www.everydayhealth.com/benzodiazepines/
Benzodiazepine Side Effects)

Benzodiazepines can cause side effects, such as:

- Drowsiness
- Dizziness
- Nausea
- Dry mouth
- Constipation
- Weight gain
- Confusion
- Trembling
- Headache
- Depression
- Changes in vision
- Worsening breathing problems
- Birth defects if taken during pregnancy

As you can see, this is just the start of a list on the terrible things that could go wrong. We were never told about any of the side effects, and the possibility of a hellish withdrawal if we ever needed to come off of it. Here is an overview of Benzodiazepine Withdrawal Syndrome

From the website:

http://www.benzo.org.uk/vernon.htm,

a doctor named Dr. Vernon Coleman who is well aware of the faults of the medical community in overprescribing and non-informing related to these awful drugs shares these facts:

Benzodiazepine   Tranquillisers
Quotations from The Drugs Myth, 1992 Dr Vernon Coleman, MB, ChB, DSc (Hon)

- In the 1960s and 1970s when the dangers associated with the barbiturates had become widely known, a newly discovered group of drugs – the benzodiazepines – were introduced as safe, effective and non addictive alternatives for patients who needed help to relax or to get to sleep. Within a very short space of time thousands of doctors were prescribing vast quantities of the benzodiazepines for millions of patients and by the late 1980s virtually every developed country in the world had a major benzodiazepine addiction problem. For the third time in less than a century doctors and the drug industry had successfully created and promoted drug addiction.
- Drugs such as heroin and cocaine are usually put into the first group whereas drugs such as the benzodiazepines inevitably find themselves in the second group. This sort of classification has no basis in science, for the benzodiazepine tranquillisers are much more

30

dangerous and much more addictive than the so called 'hard' drugs.

And, of course, whether an individual becomes an addict through his own poor choices, through ill luck or through the errors of a physician, he will still be regarded as an addict. The stigma is the same. Millions of individuals who have become hooked through absolutely no fault of their own are treated badly by doctors, by society and by employers. During the last two decades I have received tens of thousands of letters from people whose lives have been ruined (in every possible sense of the word) because of benzodiazepine addiction. Most report that the agony of their addiction has been compounded by the feelings of shame and guilt they have been encouraged to bear, and by the sense of outrage they feel at the way they have been treated.

- One of the classic ways of acquiring a drug market is to give away free supplies of a drug to non-users who try the free sample, like it and then have to pay for their supplies. This technique is regularly used by professional drug pushers. Incidentally, shortly after the benzodiazepines were first introduced into Britain supplies were donated free to hospitals in order to calm government anxieties about the cost. This mass marketing programme must surely have helped lead to the massive addiction problem which now exists.
- The benzodiazepines are probably the most addictive drugs ever created and the vast army

of enthusiastic doctors who prescribed these drugs by the tonne have created the world's largest drug addiction problem. I am well aware of the size of this problem because I have been campaigning to persuade politicians and doctors to control the benzodiazepines more effectively for most of my professional life; during that time I have heard from and spoken to tens of thousands of addicts whose lives have been ruined by these drugs.

- When patients are taken off benzodiazepines successfully, many of them say that they feel better than they have felt for years, without any further treatment. The danger of the benzodiazepines is insidious. These drugs have withdrawal effects very similar to those of barbiturates and alcohol but these withdrawal effects may take much longer to come on.

- It was known long before this that the benzodiazepines caused problems. The first scientific paper showing that they could be addictive was published in 1961 – just a year after chlordiazepoxide (the first of the benzodiazepines) had been launched in America. The first clinical report I have been able to find that detailed the addictive qualities of the benzodiazepines was published in a journal called Psychopharmacologia. It was written by three doctors from the Veterans' Administration Hospital in Palo Alto, California. The paper was entitled *Withdrawal Reactions from Chlordiazepoxide* and it described in dramatic detail how patients who had been taking the drug suffered from withdrawal symptoms when the drug was stopped.

The authors of the paper published in Psychopharmacologia described how eleven patients who had been taking fairly high doses of chlordiazepoxide for up to six months were suddenly taken off their pills and given sugar tablets instead. Ten of the eleven patients experienced new symptoms after withdrawal. Six patients became depressed, five were agitated and unable to sleep. Two of the patients had major convulsions or fits. Most of the symptoms developed within two to nine days after the drug was stopped. By the early 1970s a number of other papers had been published showing that the benzodiazepines could cause addiction. In 1975 the International Journal of the Addictions carried a major article entitled *Misuse and Abuse of Diazepam: An Increasingly Common Medical Problem.*

Over the following years I wrote dozens of newspaper and magazine articles on the subject of benzodiazepine addiction and I helped to make scores of television and radio programmes. As a result I received tens of thousands of letters from tranquilliser users (at one time 1 was getting well over a thousand letters a week from people who were hooked on tranquillisers and who wanted help). By the early 1980s I estimated that there were between two-and-a-half and three million benzodiazepine addicts in Britain – and millions more around the world. In addition to the letters from patients I also received a vast number of letters from doctors, for although tens of thousands of doctors were still handing out benzodiazepines freely a growing number were becoming aware of the problem. Many consultants and general practitioners wrote to tell me that they thought that the benzodiazepines were the most addictive drugs in common use and countless drug experts told me that in their experience patients found it far harder to get off the benzodiazepines than off any illegal drugs.

- Eventually, in January 1988 the Committee on Safety of Medicines finally issued a warning headed 'Benzodiazepine dependence and withdrawal symptoms'. The warning advised doctors that the benzodiazepines should not be used for more than four weeks, and warned that long-term chronic use was not recommended.

By then it was too late for millions of patients. The government, the drug industry and the medical profession should have acted fifteen years earlier – when the evidence they needed was first made available. The medical profession had created the biggest drug addiction problem to originate in the twentieth century. Sadly, even today, three years after that official announcement, I am still getting letters every day from British patients who are being given benzodiazepine tranquillisers and translations of my articles and books about benzodiazepines have shown that the benzodiazepine problem is only just emerging in many other countries.

- Most alarming of all, perhaps, is the fact that the medical profession, the politicians and the drug companies seem to have learned little or nothing from the tragic benzodiazepine story.

- I firmly believe that any drug prescribed for anxiety will eventually prove to be addictive, but it seems to me that neither doctors nor drug companies are prepared to abandon the search for a profitable pharmacological solution to anxiety. The result is, I fear, that in the future the problems associated with the benzodiazepines will be repeated time and time again. The benzodiazepines have caused infinitely more sorrow and despair than all illegal drugs put together and yet governments and legislators have been so busy concentrating on the control of illegal drugs such as heroin, cocaine and cannabis that they have consistently failed to act and protect patients until enormous amounts of unnecessary damage have been done. Effective controls on the barbiturates came a decade too late and the significant warning about the benzodiazepines also came well over a decade too late. Politicians and legislators have presumably assumed that because a drug is available on prescription it must be safe. If they had put one per cent of the effort that has gone into an attempt to halt illegal drug smuggling into controlling the promotion and prescribing of the benzodiazepines the public would have benefited beyond all measure.

On the same website page, Dr. Vernon Coleman continues:

The Nightmare Pills – How Millions are Caught in the Tranquilliser Trap: The latest confidential statistics from the Department of Health and Social Security show that in the last 12 months for which figures are available about 30 million prescriptions were written for tranquillisers such as Valium, Librium and Ativan.

It is easy enough to explain why doctors started prescribing tranquillisers 20 or 30 years ago. At the time they seemed a perfect answer. Barbiturates were going out of fashion. And doctors were beginning to recognise that stress related diseases are common. Tranquillisers such as Valium seemed to offer a safe solution. But it is more difficult to explain just why doctors continue to prescribe these drugs today.

For the surprising fact is that for some time now the drug companies have been warning doctors that they are NOT suitable for long-term use. My own estimate – which has not been disputed by anyone from the medical profession, the DHSS or the Home Office, is that there are about 2,500,000 tranquillisers users in Britain.

And many say they are just as difficult to come off as heroin. Joseph Tutt is not the only patient who is so angry that he is suing his doctor.

Two other readers of mine have already consulted solicitors and begun legal action. And dozens more have written to tell me that they are planning legal action.

If Tutt is successful many patients who have been given tranquillisers or sleeping tablets and whose lives have been devastated or damaged in some way could have begun proceedings within months. And it will be their doctors they will sue, not the drug companies. Some ten or fifteen years ago the drug companies were promoting products of this type with unqualified enthusiasm.

And doctors could hardly be blamed for believing that these drugs were both effective and safe. But for years now there has been no such excuse.

Drug companies making these products constantly warn doctors not to allow patients to take them for more than a week or two. They advise doctors not to make these drugs available on 'repeat prescription'. Evidence showing that these drugs are addictive and potentially dangerous has been accumulating rapidly since the early 1970s. Numerous research papers have been published showing that products in this group can cause problems such as memory loss as well as anxiety, depression and sleeplessness.

Ironically, these are the three symptoms for which they are most commonly prescribed. The Committee on Safety of Medicines has received reports showing that these drugs are well known to cause well over 100 different side effects. Earlier this month the DHSS and the Home Office publicly admitted that the size of Britain's tranquilliser addiction problem is worrying them by bringing these drugs under the Misuse of Drugs Act 1971 – the same legislation that controls drugs such as heroin. And yet thousands of doctors don't seem to take any notice. It may be true that many still don't know what else to do for patients who are suffering from anxiety or stress-related diseases. The only conclusion I can draw is that several thousand British doctors do not read articles in the medical journals nor do they study literature which is published by the drug companies.

These painfully ignorant doctors have between them created the biggest drug addiction problem this country has ever known. It's their addiction to prescribing these terrible drugs that has given us a nation of junkies. If Mr Tutt – and others like him – win, the medical profession could be facing several million very expensive lawsuits and its biggest crisis in modern history. The flood gates will have opened. Dr Coleman is the author of over 30 books including Addicts and Addictions. The paperback edition of his latest book. Life Without Tranquillisers, was published two months ago. Since then he has received more than 6,000 letters from users who, he says, are angry enough to sue the doctors that put them on the road to addiction. – Today, May 7, 1986

The upshot is that the information has been out there for years, and it is just a tragedy that we patients have not been told of the grave dangers of the hellish drugs of benzodiazepines (and anti-psychotics like Seroquel) by the medical establishment.

Chapter 4: You MUST Taper the Doses

The way you will someday be "Benzo-free" and "Seroquel-free" is to SLOWLY taper off the drugs. COLD TURKEY DOES NOT WORK! Please don't try to abruptly quit. It is a natural reaction to just flush all the pills down the toilet after realizing that they are terrible horrible "medicines" and are destroying your mind and body. But if you try to quit abruptly, you will bring on such an intense withdrawal episode that you may jump off the nearest bridge, walk into traffic, or become psychotic if you quit cold turkey. This is especially true if you have been taking them for an extended period.

Just accept that your normal sleep/wake cycle is going to be destroyed...possibly for a long time. Just concede that you will have to suffer somewhat. The key is to minimize that suffering enough so you won't give up on getting off the meds due to severe withdrawal symptoms. That means you will be needing a job or routine that forces you on a schedule. If you are not working, then you would need something to occupy your time so that you are not wishing to escape and take another pill.

Ideally, you would do this under the care of a physician. But wait? Isn't going to a doctor in the first place the reason why you got hooked onto these poisonous drugs? However, you are going to need access to a steady supply of these medications, in order to develop a long tapering schedule. Maybe work with an addiction specialist doctor who has experience with Benzodiazepine Withdrawal Syndrome.

There are so many reasons tapering is the only way to go, so please avoid the needless frustration and agony trying to go cold turkey. Just taper. Just do it! If you don't you WILL relapse over and over, or you may have a seizure and DIE, or you will suffer to the point where you will pick up a gun and point it at your head.

Either with a physician or by yourself, write down on a calendar your tapering schedule. There are many suggestions to be found from people who have done it successfully in the past. Try to make the taper as slow as you can tolerate. And keep an accurate accounting. The speed of the taper will be equivalent to how long you were on either Seroquel or Benzos (short for Benzodiazepines) and what the dosage was.

Chapter 5: Don't Worry About the Time Span

Now that you have wisely chosen to taper, it is important to point out that you should not worry about how slow the taper is. Too much people want to pick a taper that is too fast. That was my problem. I wanted that poison out of my body...and fast. I had so many false starts it is embarrassing to think about. It is understandable for people to think this way (of cutting the dosage as fast as you can). However, it is the wrong way of thinking. If you pick too fast of a taper, the odds are very very high that you fail catastrophically and you will relapse/return to the maximum dose (pre-withdrawal symptoms). The point is to be eventually free of the war prison that is Benzodiazepines (and/or Seroquel). Trying to accomplish an extremely difficult task in a hurry will only result in failure. And a loss of precious time...

On the Internet, please Google an expert who utilizes a "water titration method" named Dr. Heather Ashton. She is a leader in this field of study, and many have been helped by her work. The web site is:

http://www.benzo.org.uk/manual/

She has been so successful in helping others rid themselves of the deadly drug, so please use her guide as a tool to help you to succeed.

After many many false starts, I realized that one of my biggest mistakes was cutting too fast the doses. Therefore, I simply just kept on doing slower and slower tapers until I was able to withstand the painful effects. Thus, I just kept cutting the doses every week until I had just a negligible amount. Like I said, the LONGER your tapering schedule, the HIGHER are the odds of success. Looking back, I personally was on such a high dose of the Benzos (equivalent to 30 Valium per day), that I needed a tapering schedule that lasted over a year!

The same was true for my getting off of Seroquel. LONG, SLOW tapers was the key component to be able to endure the crazy withdrawal symptoms. There are many other things you can do to help yourself succeed in getting off of these poisons, which we will cover in later chapters. Remember always the key is that if you taper too quickly, then the withdrawal symptoms will be far too difficult to endure. Finally, keep in mind that there are individual physiological components which would surely affect how the drug is taking effect. Unfortunately, you cannot predict before what you will be feeling, but please just be ready for anything. Do NOT concern yourself with the time span until you are not taking the drugs anymore. Concern yourself with the likelihood of eventual success.

Chapter 6: Know Your Enemy

It seems that we should take a chapter to go over all the common withdrawal symptoms you may experience. We discussed many before, but here is a comprehensive list for both Seroquel and benzodiazepines. (Note: With the lists so endless, is there any wonder the drugs are so harmful? You have to ask yourself if the government is aware of such devastating withdrawal symptoms, why are the drugs still legal?)

The following is from the Seroquel related website:

http://mentalhealthdaily.com/2014/05/20/seroquel-quetiapine-withdrawal-symptoms-how-long-do-they-last/

Seroquel Withdrawal Symptoms: List of Possibilities

Below are a list of common symptoms that have been reported during Seroquel withdrawal. Keep these symptoms in mind when you come off of the medication so that you know what to expect. Although you may not experience every symptom on the list, it is likely that you will experience something when you quit taking this drug.

- **Agitation**: If you feel especially agitated, it's because you're brain is no longer receiving the drug. This drug helps many people stay calm and reduces agitation. When a person quits taking it, they may become increasingly agitated and it may last for awhile.

- **Anxiety**: In many cases this drug helps people with anxiety. When you stop taking it, your anxiety may skyrocket. Everything you do may provoke nervousness and intense anxiety. Try to realize that it is just from withdrawal and that you will recover.
- **Concentration problems**: Although this drug can cause concentration problems while you take it, you may also experience poor concentration when you stop it. Some people call this "brain fog" or foggy thinking – it is due to the fact that your brain is trying to readjust itself.
- **Depression**: When withdrawing from this antipsychotic you may spiral into deep depression. Any medication that affects neurotransmitters can result in depression when you withdraw – especially if it had a subtle antidepressant effect when you took it.
- **Dizziness**: A common withdrawal symptom from any psychiatric medication is dizziness. This may be extreme when you quit taking Seroquel, but shouldn't last longer than a few months. For most people, this sensation goes away after a few weeks, but for some, the dizziness persists for a long time. Don't freak out if the dizziness lasts longer than you anticipated – realize that it is a result of post-acute withdrawal.
- **Fatigue**: Feeling excessively lethargic, tired, and fatigued is common when quitting an antipsychotic. Although this medication tends to be sedating while you take it, the withdrawal takes a toll on overall energy levels. When your brain is trying to readjust, you may become extremely tired and feel like sleeping all day.

- **Headaches**: It is common to experience headaches when you quit taking Seroquel. The headaches may be minor or may feel like full blown migraines. These will subside eventually, but may last weeks before they go away.
- **Heart rate changes**: You may notice that your heart rate becomes excessive when you quit this drug. Some people notice that their heart beats excessively fast when they withdraw. You may also notice heart palpitations – these are caused by both withdrawal and anxiety.
- **Hypersensitivity**: A person may become hypersensitive to sights and sounds when they come off of this medication. The person may not realize that it is from drug withdrawal and their neurotransmitters are not functioning properly. Therefore normal sounds may sound excessively loud and normal sights may appear excessively bright.
- **Insomnia**: It is common to experience insomnia when you quit this drug. Insomnia is usually caused by anxiety and/or sleep disruptions. Your entire sleep cycle may be thrown off when you quit this drug and you may experience increased anxiety.
- **Irritability**: Don't be surprised if you become increasingly irritable and difficult when you stop this drug. In general the medication tends to calm people down almost to the point of a stupor. If you feel excessively irritable, know that it's likely a result of withdrawal.
- **Itching**: Some people notice when they quit this drug that they become itchy all over. If you are experiencing excessive itchiness when you stop Seroquel, just know that it's a result of

withdrawal. If it becomes too unbearable, you may want to conduct a slower taper.

- **Mood swings**: It is common to experience mood swings when you quit this drug – even if you are not bipolar. The mood swings may be more pronounced and uncontrollable if you are bipolar, but even individuals that aren't will notice that they may feel angry one minute and hopeful the next.

- **Nausea**: One of the most common symptoms associated with withdrawal from Seroquel is that of nausea. You may feel nauseated for an extended period of time until your body becomes used to functioning without the drug.

- **Psychosis**: It has been discovered that withdrawal from antipsychotics can cause psychosis. In other words, you may experience hallucinations, delusions, etc. when you are coming off of this medication. Most people don't experience psychosis when they withdraw unless they have pre-existing schizophrenia – but it is still a possibility.

- **Sleep problems**: A person may notice major changes in their sleep patterns and length when they quit taking this medication. One minute the person may have bouts of extreme insomnia and the next minute they may feel extremely tired.

- **Suicidal thoughts**: Many people take this medication to help with suicidal thoughts and depression. When you quit taking it, you may feel more suicidal than you have ever felt. This is due to the fact that your neurotransmitter levels are out of balance and you are no longer receiving the drug to help.

- **Sweating**: A very common symptom is that of profuse sweating when you stop taking Seroquel. This may be prevalent throughout the day and/or may occur while you are sleeping. You may wake up from sleep in a pool of sweat. Just know that this is your body's response to withdrawing from the drug.
- **Vision changes**: Some people experience pain in the eye and visual disturbances as a result of taking this medication. It has been hypothesized that this and other antipsychotics could lead a person to experience blurred vision even when withdrawing. Some even hypothesize potential "eye damage" as a result of taking this medication.
- **Vomiting**: Unfortunately you may vomit a lot when you stop taking Seroquel. This can be a result of intense nausea and/or your body's way of detoxifying itself. If you feel like vomiting, just know that many people experience this during withdrawal.

Note: It is documented that Seroquel stays in your system for around 1.6 days after you stop taking it. Once the drug is out of your system, it can take a long time for your neurophysiology to recalibrate itself back to homeostatic functioning.

For the withdrawal symptoms of benzodiazepines, the list is similar but so numerous it is shocking. From the website Wikipedia:

https://en.wikipedia.org/wiki/Benzodiazepine_withdrawal_syndrome

- Aches and pains[35]

- Agitation and restlessness[35]
- Akathisia
- Anxiety, possible terror and panic attacks[1][35]
- Blurred vision[35]
- Chest pain[35]
- Depersonalization[36]
- Depression (can be severe),[37] possible suicidal ideation
- Derealisation (feelings of unreality)[38]
- Diarrhea
- Dilated pupils[21]
- Dizziness[35]
- Double vision
- Dry mouth[35]
- Dysphoria[39][40]
- Electric shock sensations[4][41]
- Elevation in blood pressure[42]
- Fatigue and weakness[35]
- Flu-like symptoms[35]
- gastrointestinal problems [43][43][44]
- Hearing impairment[35]
- Headache[1]
- Hot and cold spells[35]
- Hyperosmia[45]
- Hypertension[46]
- Hypnagogia-hallucinations[16]
- Hypochondriasis[35]
- Increased sensitivity to touch[38]
- Increased sensitivity to sound[35]
- Increased urinary frequency[35]
- Indecision[35]
- Insomnia[47]
- Impaired concentration[1]
- Impaired memory and concentration[35]
- Loss of appetite and weight loss[48]
- Metallic taste[45]

- Mild to moderate Aphasia[45]
- Mood swings[35]
- Muscular spasms, cramps or fasciculations[49]
- Nausea and vomiting[47]
- Nightmares[47]
- Numbness and tingling[35]
- Obsessive compulsive disorder[50][51]
- Paraesthesia[38][45]
- Paranoia[45]
- Perception that stationary objects are moving[38]
- Perspiration[1]
- Photophobia[45]
- Postural hypotension[47]
- REM sleep rebound[52]
- Restless legs syndrome[23]
- Sounds louder than usual[38]
- Stiffness[35]
- Taste and smell disturbances[35]
- Tachycardia[53]
- Tinnitus[54]
- Tremor[55][56]
- Visual disturbances

Rapid discontinuation may result in a more serious syndrome

- Catatonia, which may result in death[57][58][59]
- Confusion[60]
- Convulsions, which may result in death[61][62]
- Coma[63] (rare)
- Delirium tremens[64][65][65]
- Delusions[66]
- Hallucinations
- Hyperthermia[47]
- homicidal ideations[67]

- Mania[68][69]
- Neuroleptic malignant syndrome-like event[70][71] (rare)
- Organic brain syndrome[72]
- Post-traumatic stress disorder[23]
- Psychosis[73][74]
- Suicidal ideation[75]
- Suicide[2][27][76]
- Urges to shout, throw, break things or harm someone[35]
- Violence[77]

As withdrawal progresses, patients often find their physical and mental health improves with improved mood and improved cognition.

Chapter 7: Don't Increase the Dosage

Absolutely the hardest part of the withdrawal symptoms (whatever they may be), is to resist the urge to increase the dosage during the tapering process. You will have so many bad days in addition to your good days. The problem is that many people (during their worst days), increase the dosage for that day. This is a bad idea. It is better to stay strong and resist the urge to increase the dose. You need your body to ADAPT slowly to ever decreasing dosages. If you waver, you will be back to square one! You will have had to start ALL OVER AGAIN, and you will have wasted time as well. Plus, you will make the entire process of early suffering that you already surmounted come back all over again. Therefore, the key is to come up with a realistic SLOW taper from the very beginning. Once started, you need to absolutely resist returning to any higher dosages you have already overcome.

The best decision is to force yourself at all costs to adhere to the tapering schedule you and your doctor agreed to. You now decided on the road back to freedom from these poisons, so try not to backtrack. Too many people start on a successful tapering program, but whenever another painful moment arrives, they will go back to their previous original dosages. They become frustrated, and they may give up hope.

Hang in there! Bear with the fact that one of the hardest things about the Benzo Withdrawal Syndrome and Seroquel Withdrawal is that it is so protracted. The withdrawal symptoms are very very bad one day, and the next two days may be almost bearable to you. Then, the next three days may feel like you are thrown into a house of torture. It is important to recognize this, and brace yourself to be strong in the face of severe adversity.

Many times during your recovery phase, it is going to feel like it will NEVER get any better. Benzo Withdrawal Syndrome is sort of like having a really bad cold that seems to never go away. Therefore, is there any wonder as to why so many give up and go back on these toxic medications? This is when you need to pick yourself up and power through it. I can promise you that it DOES get better, so keep the faith and never let go of hope.

I confess that I stumbled myself a few times too! But what is important is that I never gave up, and with each attempt it got easier and easier. Now, it has been many many years since I even had a craving for a benzodiazepine or a Seroquel tablet. And my body feels better than ever.

Chapter 8: Drink a Lot of Fluids and Eat Well

I want to include a short chapter about the need to consume ample amounts of liquid and eat a very healthy diet. For some reason it really helped me to be able to have many nutritional juices in the house. Having these withdrawal symptoms are very much like having a terrible cold. Therefore, you will need to be well hydrated and you must take care to eat well. You will need every last ounce of strength and good health to make it through this. Specific to myself, I discovered that when I am feeling stronger physically, I can better achieve my own psychological health. Drinking plenty of fluids will also help to cleanse the body too.

I went to the grocery store and bought so many fruit juices. Pomegranate, carrot, grapefruit, every possible juice felt great. I also drank a lot of chamomile tea. It is scientifically proven to help with sleep, which is a major concern for those going through withdrawal. After all, insomnia is very painful. The military tortures prisoners by withholding sleep.

I also bought a juicer and made my own smoothies too. When all natural vitamins enter your body, you strengthen your body so it can withstand the withdrawal symptoms. More and more juices will succeed in the cleansing of your circulatory system. Also, eating well within a well balanced diet will keep your body strong, and that helps you to summon the strength when you are at your wits end. Also, being healthy will give you strength to get up and do things…instead of just laying in bed all day wishing you were dead. Please keep this in mind during your road to progress.

Please make absolutely sure that you don't start substituting one poison for another. Absolutely avoid alcohol. First of all, I am writing about how to make sure your body is in 100% top shape. Don't think that alcohol will help you relax or give you more sleep. I tried that a few times with catastrophic failure. Drinking glasses of wine to try to sleep will only result in non-restful "sleep" and you will absolutely feel worse than if you drank no alcohol.

Chapter 9: Keep a Detailed Record of Your Progress

Records could be kept in many ways, but the key is to start keeping notes from day one. In this way, you will be encouraged by the small victories. You can then read about how you are getting better over long periods. Without this keeping of records, then there will be many days that frustrate you, and you won't even realize you are getting better. If you don't believe you are making progress, you will jump back to the Benzos. However, if you kept up to date very accurate journals, and detail all the days that you are triumphant, then you can be encouraged more as time goes on.I cannot say enough about keeping a record of your success, because this is a marathon, not a sprint. As the days drag on, without a clear record that you are making progress, there will be way too many times you will throw in the towel. After doing well for awhile, something may happen in your life that really stresses you out. Since the fix is so easy (just putting a pill in your mouth), you will succumb to that choice again and again.

One way would be to get another calendar (or print one out) and put it clearly where you can see it. Every day you successfully complete your tapering program, you put a big black X on that square, and just watch those days pass by. Once you have say...six weeks...full of X's, then it will be harder for you to give in when faced with a tough day.

You will feel like you have already endured so much and overcome such hardship, it will give you strength to prevent a relapse to a higher dose when you see all the progress you have made.

Chapter 10: A Tip on Xanax

Key point is to make sure that if you start with Xanax as your addiction, be aware that the withdrawal symptoms are by far the most intense and come on the fastest of all the benzos. Xanax is the shortest acting of the benzos, so it is also processed by your body and gone most rapidly. The issue with this is that the withdrawal symptoms will come on the fastest and be the most intense.

For the withdrawal process, ask your doctor to change you to one of the longer lasting Benzos like Diazepam/Valium. This will make the removal of the drug from your system slower and more gradual. This allows you to have a less painful withdrawal process.

Of course, it is important to recognize that the withdrawal will still be uber painful, but much less so because of the chemistry of the longer lasting benzodiazepines. The withdrawal will be smoother, and some of the most awful symptoms like those electrical jolts that feel like a seizure, will likely be absent.

Chapter 11: Be Active in an Internet Support Group

When you are attempting to face the most challenging task in your life, it makes it easier if you feel that there are others who commiserate and understand. That is why getting involved and active with others who are having similar symptoms is so critical and valuable. When I was in the depths of despair and suffering from the physical and mental symptoms, I found that constant reading of other people's misfortunes and sufferings served me well. Communicating with others on an Internet chatroom and blog (about the withdrawal process) were a saving grace for me. We would commiserate with each other, and encourage each other.

It is so clear that when you feel you are suffering all alone, it is so much harder to endure what you are going through. However, if you are knowing that there are so many people trying to endure what you are grappling with, it becomes so much easier to push through what you have to overcome as well.

Start with http://www.benzosupport.org/ as a good place to start.

Here is another: http://www.drugs.com/answers/support-group/benzodiazepine-withdrawal/

And another: http://www.benzobuddies.org/forum/

Finally, one more: http://www.mdjunction.com/benzodiazepine-withdrawal

There may be a local chapter already in existence where you can physically travel to, like NA (Narcotics Anonymous) or AA (Alcoholics Anonymous). That would be very useful and ideal. However, there are so many more in existence on the World Wide Web. The whole point is to make sure that you don't suffer by yourself. If you think you are the only one suffering, then surely you will relapse over and over forever. Being with others who are enduring the same thing that you are going through will vastly increase the chances that you will make it. People suffering together lean on each other and give each other support and encouragement.

The more time you spend reading others' stories, taking their advice, writing and sharing your own struggles, you will have more support to lean on during times of maximum pain. Being in a community will become a source of strength you can rely on when the cravings become the strongest.

Chapter 12: Don't Become Frustrated

You may, just like I did, have a dozen "relapses" where you go back on the poisons of Seroquel and Benzodiazepines (Please note though that I was on one of the highest doses of benzos and Seroquel, and for a very long time period). The important point I want to emphasize here is that you cannot let yourself become frustrated and give up! Remember, you CAN and WILL get there. As I shared, I was taking two 5 mg tabs of Valium, two 2 mg tabs of Xanax, and two 2 mg tabs of Klonopin, ALL AT ONCE every single night and even occasionally mixed alcohol with it! It was a deadly combination, and one of the highest doses that anyone has ever taken and survived to taper successfully from (according to a few addiction doctors that I dealt with)!

It is so easy to give up because the poison has such a hold on us. Some of the most precious things we need, like the need to become calm, and our sleep, is taken away during the Benzo Withdrawal Syndrome and the Seroquel Syndrome.

Here are some tips on combating frustration from the Positivity Blog:

http://www.positivityblog.com/index.php/2015/06/04/overcome-frustration/

Step 1: Be here now.

When you are frustrated then you are often somewhere in the future in your mind. Somewhere you wish you would be. Or you are reliving a stumble or failure from your past.

Snap out of those headspaces and calm down by focusing your mind and attention on what is now, right here at this moment.

You can do so by for example:

- **Focusing on your breathing.** Sit down, close your eyes and just focus on the air going and out of your nose for 1-2 minutes. Take calm and slightly deeper breaths than usual and breathe with your belly and not your chest.
- **Focus on what is around you at this time.** The sun shining in through your window. The kids playing out in the street and the cars and people going by. The smells and feeling of the clothes and warmth of the sun on your skin. Do this for 1-2 minutes to get your attention back to the present moment.

Step 2: Appreciate what you do have.

After you have pulled your attention back to where it can be most helpful focus it on what is still positive in your life.

The quickest and easiest way to do so is to focus it on appreciating what you do have.

A favorite of mine during this step is the important things we may sometimes take for granted. Like for instance:

- A warm home and a roof over your head.

- Plenty of drinkable water.
- Not having to go hungry.
- Access to the internet.
- Your friends and family.

Spend a few minutes on this and you'll find much to be grateful for.

Step 3: Focus on what you can do right now.

With your attention in the present moment and your mood a more grateful and positive one it is now time to get constructive about what frustrates you.

You can do that by asking yourself:

What is one small step I can take right now to improve this situation?

It may be to see what you can learn from what frustrates you and to try another path towards your goal.

Or it could be to try one more time and to keep going (because not all things in life will come to you the first, second or third time you try).

Or it could be you simply realizing that you may have taken on a bit much lately or things have been tough and that you need to take this evening or a few days to just relax, take care of yourself and perhaps simplify a bit.

So that you can recharge and then get back into moving towards what you want out of your life in a more focused way.

The point is that you will hit maximum frustration a million times on Benzodiazepine Withdrawal/Seroquel withdrawal. They are among the most difficult drugs to get over in this life. As I wrote, many have said that getting off of them is harder than getting off of cocaine or heroin!

Read the article: "Valium can be harder to withdraw than from heroin"

http://www.vice.com/read/valium-can-be-harder-to-withdraw-from-than-heroin

Also there is this: "Benzo withdrawal vs. Heroin withdrawal

http://www.bluelight.org/vb/threads/527472-Benzo-withdrawal-vs-heroin-withdrawal

And finally consider this website referring to how benzodiazepines are far more of a danger than heroin in America today:

http://worsethanheroin.com/

Getting off of Benzodiazepines will be one of the most difficult things you can ever experience, and being accepting of what you are going to have to endure can help empower you. Just imagine yourself someday off Benzodiazepines, like me. Then you can feel so good that the fight you are fighting is worth it. You will feel so much better as a result of being finally off these poisons that the feeling of liberation will make all the frustration that you endured worth it in the end.

Chapter 13: Timeline For the Withdrawal Period

This is related to the last chapter is the sense that if you really understand the extensive timeframe of the withdrawal period, you will become less frustrated (and less often). Here is where it gets tough to admit...at least for me. After nearly TEN YEARS after I started to withdraw from Benzos/Seroquel, I am STILL feeling mild effects. These effects center on my being unable to fall asleep easily at night.

In my distant past before I even touched these poisons, I could fall asleep nearly instantly. Nearly every night, when my head hit the pillow, I could sleep within five minutes and I was very groggy when I woke up. I could take a nap even during the daytime! I was truly a deep sleeper. After my horrible experience on Benzos and Seroquel, I often yearn for being able to sleep so easily and soundly.

But perhaps, at least for me, it was a partial blessing that I am not chronically tired and sleeping all the time. But, it still sucks not to be able to sleep whenever and wherever you want in an instant.

Therefore, what I am trying to say is that just be ready to experience withdrawal symptoms for many months, if not years. However, IT DOES GET BETTER GRADUALLY! The timeline for YOU will be truly completely unpredictable.

Much will depend on how long you have been taking either medication. Some can fully recover from the symptoms within a month or so, but others may battle with symptoms for months or years! Since I was abusing the drugs at the maximum level, I should have expected the longest of recovery periods.

Still, I feel so amazing being off of those poisonous drugs. I feel having the determination and finally ridding myself of all those drugs was the single greatest accomplishment of my entire life!

I would like to say as a general rule that some sources I read about on my research suggests that it would take at least 90 days for you to see any kind of improvement. We have been shredded with the worst of the worst drugs, so please lower your expectations and prepare yourself for a VERY long recovery period.

Who knows, if by chance you recover fully within a week or a month, you have been luckier than nearly everyone. That may be the case, especially if you have not taken the drugs for an extended period of time.

As I shared, I had been taking very very high doses for at least six long years, so it took my brain and body at least that long to get most of my symptoms to disappear.

Chapter 14: Take Care of Your Body

To make sure you maximize your chances of success (with the fewest number of relapses), please take care of your body. As a general rule, when your body is the strongest, you can overcome struggles easier. This is true of both mental and physical trials. Benzodiazepine and Seroquel withdrawal involve both, and it would be wise to try and maintain your health at its maximum. The absolute worst thing you can do (and I learned from experience), is just sit there suffering and wallow in your miserable symptoms. Lying in bed all day just makes a bad situation even worse. If you do this, all your mind will think about is how horrible you feel, and when you should buckle and take previous higher doses of pills.

Therefore, make sure to get up and take showers and exercise. Or go outside and do things that strengthen your physical health. If you just retreat to your bedroom and stare at the clock, the recovery period of say three months will seem like three decades. Plus, just being immobile will make you even more physically sick. Then, it would be impossible to last through until the symptoms begin to abate.

You have to make sure your body is in tip top shape through your ordeal, because you are going to need strength to fight. If you are physically feeling weak and helpless, it will be an impossible task to overcome the periods of time when the craving for the drugs will be at its maximum. Join a gym or spa, and take to nature walks in your favorite forest preserve. The healthier your body is, the faster it can get rid of all the toxins and damage that the drugs inflicted.

When I finally recovered, I found that going to the gym once a day (or exercising at home) was instrumental in my continued recovery. Also, always eating a well balanced meal full of good nutritional food was pivotal. Once you build up your body, you can feel more confident in yourself too, and with that confidence comes the energy and strength to push through when you are in your worst periods.

Chapter 15: Give Tapering Doses Away

This is very very important. After you determine your proper tapering schedule, you must give the drugs to someone else who will give them to you on the correct schedule. They can live in the same house as you, but they MUST either keep the medication in a safe or so deeply hidden that you will not be able to find the medications. If you try to self medicate, you will likely end up cheating and breaking your planned tapering schedule. And you may do this multiple times. This will result in a loss of time and much more frustration.

If you keep the medicines yourself and try to administer them yourself, what will happen is that when the withdrawal symptoms progressively get worse, you will go back to your max dose immediately, and you will be back to square one. And the nature of these demonic drugs are that you will have OK days, and then the days from Hell.

One week you may have lessened drug withdrawal symptoms, and then the following week the withdrawal symptoms will come back in a fury. You will experience possibly some of the worst symptoms ever the following week. You will think you will die. But it is within these absolutely worst moments that you must persevere. If someone else is controlling giving you the doses, it relieves that responsibility from you. You know that you will only receive the tapering dose ONCE and at a certain time of the day. You won't be reaching for it when you are hurting and take additional doses. Please please consider this valuable step in your recovery. It is crucial for your success.

Chapter 16: Withdrawal Symptoms Are Endless

It is important to recognize that there are so many withdrawal symptoms and they occur in stages. These range from acute dreaded anxiety and nervousness and chronic intractable insomnia. You may also have physical symptoms like diarrhea and nausea.

It is important to appreciate that if you have had a history of addiction in your life, then you could increase the chance of developing an addiction and the time it takes to eventually recover from it.

Note that each benzodiazepine has different half-lives. The longer the half life, the longer it will take for the withdrawal symptoms to kick in. A longer lasting drug like Valium will take a few days for the symptoms to develop while a short acting one like Xanax will cause symptoms to appear just 8-12 hours later after stopping the drug.

Here are some of the possible symptoms taken from the website:
http://americanaddictioncenters.org/benzodiazepine/length-of-withdrawal/,

Here is a listing of all the common Benzodiazepine withdrawal effects:

Anxiety, panic, insomnia, muscle spasms or tension, nausea and/or vomiting, diarrhea, blurred vision, seizures, hallucinations, short-term memory impairment, trouble concentrating, clouded thinking, mood swings, agitation, drug cravings, twitching and weight loss due to a decreased appetite.

(However, you may experience symptoms even not on this list)

For Seroquel, there is this information from the website about the withdrawal symptoms:

https://www.alternativetomeds.com/articles/seroquel-withdrawal/

Seroquel withdrawal insomnia is trademark when it comes to symptoms of discontinuing this medication, some people have even reported that months after discontinuing this drug, they still have insomnia and sleep disturbances. Some of the other symptoms include: agitation, severe restlessness, irritability, manic depression, manic excitement, restless leg syndrome, nausea, vomiting, vision problems, dizziness, rapid heart rate, hearing voices, shakes, weakness, constipation, gas, indigestion, hallucinations, delusions, stomach pain or swelling, increased appetite, excessive weight gain, headaches, pain in the joints, dry mouth, stuffy nose, decreased sexual desire, strange or unusual dreams, loss of coordination, tingling or numbness in the arms or in the legs, difficulty concentrating, difficulty speaking, difficulty thinking, breast enlargement in men, irregular menstrual cycles, and discharge from breasts.

Just understand that the withdrawal symptoms have short and long term withdrawal periods and features. The emphasis here is that there are an OCEAN of poisonous symptoms with these terrible drugs.

Chapter 17: Post Recovery Benzo/Seroquel Support

It is crucial to recognize that it is very likely that you will have problems related to your benzodiazepine and Seroquel addiction for many more years after you "recover". When you finally get to the point where you have finished your taper and are no longer taking Benzodiazepines and Seroquel, you have to recognize that you have to be on guard for the rest of your life. You must be very very guarded about relapsing. Make sure that you avoid anyone who has benzodiazepines and or Seroquel. Keep active on message boards and keep attending support groups in your area.

In addition, you must make sure that you address the mental/physical state(s) which made you seek out Seroquel or Benzodiazepines in the first place. If you are still with the boyfriend/girlfriend that made you crazy and rush off to see the doctor to get benzos and Seroquel, then you are very likely to find yourself in a situation where you may take those harmful drugs again. If you are still remaining in the job (or field of work) that gave you great psychological stress and misery, then you are inviting another episode where you may break down.

There was one support group that I attended briefly where one gentleman quoted the saying, "The one and only thing you have to change—is everything". With some exaggeration, you need to change your environment (physical and psychological), where you are in a better, safe place.

Chapter 18: Don't Forget to Pray

Alcoholics Anonymous and other support and recovery groups stress that we must submit to "a higher power" to be able to find the strength to overcome. Some may call this higher power "God", but every individual can have their own definition of who or what this higher power is.

(From Alcoholics Anonymous 12 Step Program)

2. Came to believe that a power greater than ourselves could restore us to sanity.

AA believes that people with an alcohol addiction need to look to something greater than themselves to recover. Those working the steps are free to choose whatever higher power works for them.

- Learn more about Step 2.

3. Made a decision to turn our will and our lives over to the care of God as we understood Him.

For this step, the alcoholic consciously decides to turn themselves over to whatever or whomever they believe their higher power to be. With this release often comes recovery.

When I was in my worst withdrawal moments, it gave me great solace to pray for strength. While I am Catholic, I believe it is of great benefit if one can ask God or whatever higher power they can rely on to give them the fortitude to tough it out.

Chapter 19 Consider Herbal Remedies

For my continued issues of sleep, I found it so very helpful to turn to natural herbal remedies. Some of these include Valerian Root (for sleep), Melatonin (for sleep), Lemon Extract (for sleep), and Chamomile Tea (for sleep). St. John's Wort I tried also with some success for anxiety and depression. Plus I drank Ginseng Tea as well for general well being.

There are many many other herbal natural remedies with far fewer side effects that you may try. Please research by yourself all the options out there. The possibilities are limitless.

Although it is not a natural herbal remedy, I also took some Benadryl at night to help me with sleep as well. It seemed to help me on many occasions. Experiment with all that others are sharing too in the chatrooms and forums. Your herbal solution is out there!

Herbal Remedies will not be the saving grace and make all the withdrawal symptoms disappear, but they will help you endure such a terrible horrible experience. During this time, any help will be much appreciated.

Chapter 20 Other Methods and Practices to Success

Some find it the only way to kick Benzodiazepines is to enter in an In-Patient Rehab center. A famous singer named Stevie Nicks went to an in-patient facility to kick her terrible addiction to benzos. On a website titled: "Klonopin: More Deadly Than Coke", Stevie Nicks described her ordeal as hellish, and one that could only be conquered in an in-patient facility. Here is the website where the article is located:

http://www.benzo.org.uk/nicks.htm

While not everyone can afford this kind of care, it may be worth it if you can get your health insurance to cover the stay. It may be a rather long stay, but during the first few weeks the withdrawal symptoms may be too much for you to handle at home. You may even face life threatening symptoms where you may need a doctor and medical team around (e.g. seizures). I am just throwing this suggestion out there if you have found yourself failing over and over again during the initial few weeks of the taper.

There are others who I read had moderate success with acupuncture, meditation, and Yoga as ways to cope with the terrible withdrawal symptoms. The possibilities are endless, and you should continue to search until you find some things which can help you get better. Keep being active on the message boards and group forums and try to find more ideas which will work for you. Never give up!

Conclusion

Basically, this book (meant to be a short read as an e-book) is to share my story of how I inadvertently "fell in" to probably the worst most painful experience of my life. I regret it so much but what can I do if I wallow in self pity that this happened to me? I just have to learn to live with it (the failures that resulted from the addiction to the drugs and the long term consequences of these dangerous psychoactive drugs). I remain convinced, and no one can change my mind, that there are other solutions than the ones proposed by ill-informed doctors and institutions. If you have been on one of these drugs, and wish to get off, I hope my suggestions can rid you of your plague. I pray for everyone afflicted with this curse, and I will hope that you can be successful one day as I have been. Please never give up hope. I was one of the absolute worst cases. And I survived and made it to the finish line.

Always keep in mind that the progress will be a non-linear one. One of the main reasons why recovery from benzodiazepines and Seroquel is so difficult is because the recovery process and duration is so protracted and non-linear. In other words, this is not like a cut on the leg which heals gradually and consistently over a predictable period of time. Some days and weeks will be tolerable, and other weeks it will be nearly unbearable! Not being fully aware of this made my recovery time much harder and longer than it should have been. When I was well into my taper and then it suddenly became much more painful without warning, I would give up because I did not have all the facts. Remember, I even tried initially to quit cold turkey—even on the sky high doses I was on!

If I had known that I could never hope to quit all of a sudden cold turkey, then I would have saved so much time, frustration (from relapsing to a higher earlier dose), and mental and physical suffering from guaranteed failure. If I had understood how important it was to not increase the dose, if I knew from the beginning the importance of being on support groups and keeping your body healthy, I could have recovered much sooner. I am so hoping and praying that writing down my own experience and sharing my ideas on how to be free of these psychoactive psychiatric drugs will improve the odds of success. I hope that people laboring under this condition will take some of my pearls of wisdom to make themselves better.

A few final thoughts are to avoid caffeine and sugar. A neurologist David Perlmutter, MD, on the website (http://www.benzosupport.org/Benzo.pdf), stated that people in benzodiazepine withdrawal can become hypersensitive to the stimulating effects of sugars. Instead, he recommends whole, organic foods and an intake of "adequate dietary protein" several times daily, as well as complex carbohydrates to smooth out blood sugar levels.

Please just do your best and never give up hope. You will make it. It is never too late to rid yourself of these terrible drugs. After you are fully recovered, tell everyone you know to avoid these drugs. Tell people how you managed to succeed if they are laboring under the myriad of withdrawal symptoms. Above all, don't give up imagining yourself a healthier you. This is just one more trial (albeit maybe the hardest trial) that you will have to overcome in life, and return to gratitude when you are finally off and free. Namaste...